I0778703

Table of Content

Introduction 3

What is Clean Eating and Why is it Important? 4

10 Reasons to Give Clean Eating a Try 6

7 Simple Principles and Guidelines of Clean Eating 9

15 Simple Recipes to Start Your Clean Eating Journey 11

How Does Clean Eating Aid in Maintaining Health and Managing Diseases? 14

Clean Eating 10 Day Challenge – Jump on Board – You Won't Regret It! 17

Conclusion 23

Introduction

So much emphasis with gusto has been put on eating the right kind of foods and avoiding 'bad foods'. This sort of movement has created quite a stir in many phases of dieting and the food industry with each and every one having a different definition of what clean eating is.

Either way, it all points to eating certain foods which are healthy and avoiding those categorized as 'not healthy'.

The main aim is to ensure you eat and stay healthy as a result. We are what we eat, as it goes and so it should be that we eat clean foods. Clean eating can also be called eating real foods.

When we speak about real foods, we mean foods which are as close as possible to their natural state. The shortest route of getting it to your plate is normally preferred than packaging, flavoring and coloring and all refining processes.

This ensures it is free from chemicals, unhealthy fats and all sorts of junk that can cause health problems in the long run.

In this report, clean eating has been given the center stage to create the true understanding to help you make the right food choices; know what to eat, the right amount and what you are supposed to avoid.

The guiding principles and rationale of clean eating are properly explained to you step by step. You will understand the importance of eating real foods as compared to your pizza and pasta, and why you should consider salads instead.

If you have never tried eating clean, or have no idea what it involves, then you will not worry any other time. Simple recipes that are homemade are well outlined to induct you in to clean eating.

And finally, are you ready to take on a challenge to see if you really weigh up to the matter? A comprehensive challenge is outlined for you to try. One thing to keep in mind all through is that, *natural is always better!*

What is Clean Eating and Why is it Important?

You've probably heard before about clean eating but do not exactly know what it's about and how to join the health trend. Clean eating is consuming whole foods which are near as possible to their natural state.

In other words, it is eating only foods which have undergone minimal processes of refining, processing and handling, making them as close to their natural state as possible.

It does not involve eating a specific amount of food or less of something, but being mindful of where the food comes from, its process and how you finally put it on your plate.

Nowadays, it is difficult to find foods which have not been refined or processed in some way. This becomes a challenge for clean eating enthusiasts.

The rationale of clean eating emphasizes on raw food options such as fruits and vegetables while eliminating refined grains, sugars, salt and unhealthy fats and proteins.

Should You Be Eating Clean?

Anyone aspiring for a healthy diet should go for clean foods. Eating clean is very easy to follow and does not require any strenuous effort apart from being mindful of your food choices.

Unlike dieting, you are not restricted to any specific amount of food and hence calories. You can eat as much as you would like to, or less for that matter.

What is important is to ensure that you make healthy food choices by selecting foods that are not refined or processed. Choose foods which are as close to their natural and raw state as much as possible.

How to Go about Eating Clean Food and Why it is Important to You

Clean eating has a lot of dietary benefits that comes along with it. Knowing how to make the right food choices is only the beginning. With the challenge of not knowing which food is to be considered clean, it is vital that you follow these steps to be able to eat clean.

- Eliminate processed foods: Processed foods have undergone various refining stages. They have additives and ingredients which are considered unhealthy. To begin with, check whether the ingredient list has anything that is classified as additive or artificial colors.

-

- Many refined foods have sodium, sugar and fat which do not qualify them as clean foods. There are however clean packaged foods such as whole-wheat pasta, baby spinach and chickpeas which are all good clean eating options.

- Eat more veggies: Vegetables are classy sources of vitamins A and K which help improve your vision and immune system. Go for fresh vegetables which are obtained straight from the farm, they are unprocessed and clean.

- Eat healthy fats: When eating clean, you do not need to cut back on all fat, but instead opt for clean options or healthy fats. Swap out saturated fats such as those found in meat, cheese and butter. Healthy fats are vital in improving the health of your heart and also in raising the level of the good cholesterol, HDL cholesterol.

- Reduce alcohol: This may contain unhealthy sugars and excess amount of calories which is not good for your health. Avoid mixed drinks containing lots of sugars. Be moderate in your alcohol intake-one drink per day for women and two for men.

- Monitor your salt intake: Many people have a problem of taking more than the recommended limit of 2,300 mg of sodium per day. This exposes them to high blood pressure. By eating clean, you should avoid packaged foods which are high in sodium.

- Eat whole grains: Choose whole grains which contain bran and germ, unlike refined grains which have them removed during processing. When shopping, check the label to ascertain that it is 'whole wheat' and not just 'wheat'.

- Check the portion size of meat: Eat less meat. But this does not mean that you entirely eliminate any prospect of meat. Certain meats have saturated fat which does not constitute healthy eating. Lean meat is a preferred option.

- Eat more fruits: Fruits are naturally sweet, delicious, rich in potassium and vitamin C. Take 1½ to 2 cups of fruit per day to obtain the recommended vitamins. Go for whole unprocessed fruits which are raw and obtained straight from the farm.

- Clean eating requires your deliberate effort by consciously choosing what to eat and being mindful all the time. It is not difficult once you are aware of what you should be eating and what to avoid.

- Avoid or cut back on anything refined or containing unknown ingredients which form a lengthy list on the label. These are most likely processed and ultimately unclean foods.

10 Reasons to Give Clean Eating a Try

Clean eating comes with a whole load of health benefits that will help you change your life for the better.

When you start eating clean, you make a decision to enjoy a longer healthier life, free from common ailments caused by chemicals found in most processed foods. You save yourself from medical bills as a result. On the other hand, filling your fridge with organic produce isn't expensive at all.

However, what is it about clean eating that makes it so important, and why should anyone start eating clean? Here are ten reasons why you should join this growing health trend and start eating clean.

1. You become more mindful

So many people eat in response to their cravings and appetite, but very few actually make the decision to eat consciously by selecting certain foods and ditching others. When it comes to clean eating, this is not the case. You will have to be mindful of what you decide to eat.

There are so many processed foods which are man-made, unnatural and unhealthy. If you decide to eat clean, you will opt for natural foods which are not refined or processed. This makes you a more aware of your food choices and therefore ensures improvement in your eating habits.

2. Improves your metabolism

Clean foods such as vegetables and fruits are good for boosting your metabolism. If you are planning on shedding the excess pounds, then avoid sugary and processed foods which pile the pounds. You are also likely to lose weight faster and effectively when eating clean as opposed to cheese, pasta, bread and other processed foods.

3. Improves your skin and appearance

Do you want a glowing skin that is resistant to aging? Then clean eating will make you achieve this. Eating clean foods such as fruits and vegetables helps in reducing inflammation in the skin which is brought about by consuming sugary foods. Clean eating prevents collagen in the skin from breaking down which would lead to fine lines and less glow.

4. Improves your concentration

Do you want to stay sharp and focused? You might consider eating more whole foods and avoid too much sugar. Eating processed foods has been associated with feeling foggy and unfocused because of high blood sugar which also reduces your memory. Avoid anything sugary such as bottled salad dressing or your favorite piece of cake.

5. You become more energized

Most clean foods such as fruits are guaranteed sources of instant energy whenever you feel weak or lacking energy. If you eat fruits for the afternoon, you are likely to overcome the afternoon slump and grogginess since high fiber fruits provide critical vitamins to keep you alert and energized.

6. Saves you cents

One of the perks of eating clean foods is that, you will be able to save more inadvertently. You will not fall sick often and therefore you can scrape away medical bills and use the money elsewhere.

It is cost-effective and you will be able to shop locally, being mindful about your budget and expenses. This reduces unnecessary use of money in buying spices, sugars and other refined, processed cost, so you save from all sides.

7. You will sleep better

Sleep is part of the business of staying healthy, and eating the right things has a direct bearing to the quality of sleep that you get. If you want to sleep soundly, take out the caffeine, juices and replace them with evening fruits and salads. Sleep is vitally important for your health, so eat mindfully for better sleep.

8. Reduces the risk for diabetes

Diabetes is primarily caused by consuming too much sugar and processed junk food. This multiplies your risk for diabetes and coupled with lack of exercise, there can be no way out.

To avoid this menace, you have to make clean food choices by eliminating sugar or using healthier substitutes. For example, don't go for flavored yogurt, choose plain yogurt and keep your body moving.

9. Better mood and stronger body

Do you want to feel revitalized and energized all day long? Studies have shown that people who eat less sugar are more likely to be happy and in a good mood as compared to their opposite counterparts. Eating clean has a direct relation to having better mood and a stronger body which is immune to diseases.

10. Helps you lose weight

By boosting your metabolism and reducing your cravings, clean eating is a major boost for those looking to tone down and shed the excess

pounds. If you shun processed, sugary and junk food, you will be on your way to avoiding weight gain and losing body fat.

Make a decision to change your eating habits. Opt for non-sugary, natural food options and start witnessing a positive change in your health and life in general.

Eating clean foods is more than just a dietary change; it will impact positively on your state of mind and physical well-being. Choose clean foods and start enjoying life in full gear!

7 Simple Principles and Guidelines of Clean Eating

Among nutrition scientists and health-conscious eaters, clean eating isn't just a buzz word that has been invented for the sake. It represents a lifestyle of making good food choices and following set guidelines and principles which are associated with clean eating.

Certainly, it isn't an idea that was invented yesterday, but has taken the center stage in recent times through promotion by nutritionists, fitness models and bodybuilders.

The principles of clean eating are trenchant and easy to follow and easily adaptable to any kind of lifestyle. By following them, you will be part of the new revolution that is looking to bring change in eating habits of many people. Here are the guidelines and principles for clean eating.

1. Choose whole natural foods and eliminate processed foods

One of the main guiding principles of clean eating is to go for foods that have minimal processing, or which can be obtained directly without undergoing any processing at all.

The shortest route to your plate is considered the best. Whole foods are free from additives, chemicals and flavors which are all considered to be unclean.

Most processed foods are packaged and contain lots of sugar. Be mindful of when going for them with the exception of certain packaged foods which are not processed such as packaged white rice or green beans.

2. Eat five to six portion sized meals in a day

Eating clean includes eating mindfully when it comes to portions. Do not take hefty main meals but instead six portion sized meals to keep your energy levels up. This prevents you from skimping on certain meals or even overeating in certain instances. It keeps your blood sugar levels in check for optimum performance.

3. Take exercising seriously

You do not want to eat and stay inactive. Get moving by engaging in physical activity which is important in many ways. Exercising will improve your health by improving blood circulation and you burn calories to lose weight.

4. Minimize fat, salt and sugar

When you decide to eat clean, it comes without any effort to minimize fat, salt and sugar intake. This is because by reducing processed foods, you also reduce the amount of processed sugars, sodium and unhealthy fats.

Most people find it difficult at first but then they get used to it and everything is easy. Clean foods are naturally low in sugars, fats and salts and those that have any of them becomes a healthy substitute.

5. Include healthy amounts of proteins, carbohydrates and fats

When we speak of clean eating, it does not mean typically to reduce certain essential minerals or vitamins, it only means going for the healthy options and in their right amounts.

It is vital to include protein in every meal as it is a vital energy booster and helps in building your muscles. It is also important in curbing your appetite and reducing your cravings which would otherwise lead to unhealthy eating.

6. Eat less meat

While meat is a good source of protein, iron and vitamin B12, too much of it can saturate fat and cholesterol which is unhealthy for you. This does not mean that you cut meat entirely out, but instead eat less of it to avoid piling up on saturated fat and cholesterol which could increase the risk of heart disease.

7. Eat more veggies, fruits and whole grains

Vegetables, fruits and whole grains are normally low in calories and come packed with minerals, vitamins and fiber. Incorporating them in your meals will bring the magic touch of eating clean.

It is recommended that you eat at least 2 to 3 ½ cups of fruit each day and include vegetables such as spinach. Before starting any meal, you can start off with a fruit salad or a vegetarian entrée. Whole grains are rich in fiber which makes you feel fuller for longer periods, eliminating hunger and cravings.

By following these principles and guidelines in your everyday dieting, you will experience the health benefits of clean eating.

Clean eating is a simple procedure that you can start today to have a positive lifestyle change without much effort. It is flexible and meant to help you enjoy the lifelong benefits of eating healthy.

15 Simple Recipes to Start Your Clean Eating Journey

Simple recipes that are easy to prepare are available for you when you want to start eating clean. The most important thing to remember is to go for whole foods in their natural state, and minimize on processed foods as much as possible.

Adding on to this, you can make them as stylish as you would like to with a blend of your cooking skills to bring out the whole savory taste.

Consider these simple recipes to begin your clean eating journey.

1. Quinoa Salad with Asparagus, Dates and Oranges

This is a simple recipe that you can prepare in under 20 minutes. It is packed with protein and all the essential amino acids. Rich in fiber, the whole grain quinoa is the perfect source with 5 grams of fiber per cup. This can be taken as a side dish salad.

2. Carrot soup with yogurt

Soups are a permanent mainstay when it comes to clean eating. Carrot soup with yogurt is your perfect blend, delicious, tasty and refreshing. This rich and creamy soup gives a smooth velvety richness which makes it a perfect substitute for butter.

3. Grilled chicken and vegetable quesadillas with tomatillo sauce

With lots of veggies and tomatillo sauce, this recipe is tasty and refreshing. Try it out and is very easy to prepare.

4. Oven fried sweet potatoes

Sweet potatoes are rich in beta carotene (pre-Vitamin A), Vitamin C, and potassium, not to mention fiber and complex carbohydrates, making them a better choice than white potatoes in most cases. By oven frying sweet potatoes, you cut out the calories and unhealthy fat found in them but still maintain their crispy taste.

5. Salmon and broccoli with tangy lemon sauce

Super easy and super-fast to make, this recipe is rich in omega 3 fatty acids which are a type of healthy fats, rich in protein and excellent in reducing inflammation. If you find yourself pressed for time, just prepare this and you will not miss anything. It is also rich in fiber with the broccoli and the lemon sauce for a contrasting sweet taste.

6. Carrot cake oatmeal cookies

This dessert is rich and nutritious. You can use it for the perfect aftertaste when the party is over or after dinner. The oatmeal is high in fiber and comes with a gritty taste. This recipe is rich in minerals such as potassium and vitamins which are very essential for you.

7. Arugula, grape and sunflower seed salad

This super clean salad highlights a number of fresh foods. All of them are nutritious, fresh, and unprocessed. It provides a wonderful flavor experience with sassy arugula, the sweet taste of grapes, and the salty, nutty flavor of sunflower seeds.

Even though it is a salad, it is very filling and stuffed full of vitamins, minerals, and nutrients your body needs to be healthy.

8. Vanilla almond chia breakfast pudding

This wholesome breakfast option is a combination of healthy colors that provide you with nutrients and vitamins to jump start your day. The chia seed will give you energy and act as an antioxidant at the same time. It also contains omega-3s, calcium and fiber. You will feel energized and inspired throughout your day with this recipe.

9. Roasted Shrimp and Broccoli

This dinner recipe is quick and easy to prepare, requiring only fifteen minutes of your time. Once ready, it is packed with proteins and vitamins which ensure you not only eat clean, but also get the vital minerals for your body to perform well.

10. Vegetable hash with poached eggs.

This vegetable hash can be your perfect replacement for a meatless recipe instead of pizzas or pasta. You can switch up and opt for this recipe which is going to do you good with the beautifully topped poached eggs and vegetables full of fiber to create a balanced vegetarian meal. It's easy and fast to prepare.

11. Delicious Tenderloin Steak with Marmalade Made of Red Onions

Containing simple, quality, flavorful ingredients, this recipe is packed with nutrients for clean eating. The steak is broiled to remove excess fat, and topped with delicious onions that bring a sweet and sour punch. This meal is extremely satisfying and helps you build solid muscle, while maintaining glucose levels at a healthy baseline

12. Tuna Scaloppini with onion, mint and almond topping

Once in a while, it is recommended that you should eat a variety of seafood. This recipe and its combination consist of clean eating ingredients which are healthy for you.

Tuna provides you with healthy fats such as omega-3 which acts as an antioxidant and also very rich in protein. It also boosts your immune system, lowers blood pressure and enhances your immune system. Topped with a mixture of onions, mint, and heart-healthy almonds this recipe is savory and tasty.

13. Lemony chicken kebabs with tomato-parsley salad

When wanting to eat clean, it is important to have a recipe with few recipes for keeping check and sticking to the right ingredients. This Lemony chicken kebab with tomato-parsley salad is perfect for your afternoon and consists of just six ingredients.

To begin with, marinate the chicken in the morning before prep time to make it easy for you in the afternoon. It is rich in fiber and protein and will make you feel satisfied throughout your afternoon.

14. Greek Salad with Pita Croutons

This salad will lighten up your lunch with its rich ingredients which act as anti-cancer compounds, and anti-inflammatory. It has loads of olives in it to give you healthy fats and can be combined with grain bread.

15. Kale, Quinoa and Cherry Salad

This is an easy salad for lunch and can be prepared from your leftovers. Make sure to use organic, unsalted chickpeas and organic goat cheese. It is refreshing and will power you through your afternoon.

These clean eating recipes will certainly provide you with a new dimension when choosing the right food options. They are simple, easy to prepare and come packed with nutrients, proteins, vitamins and fiber.

Choose to eat clean today, and enjoy all the benefits of staying healthy with these recipes that will make your cooking experience unforgettable.

How Does Clean Eating Aid in Maintaining Health and Managing Diseases?

Loading up your diet with clean foods is a major boost for a healthy lifestyle, and it goes a long way in ensuring you enjoy a longer life while staying away from the doctor. But what does clean eating really do to maintain your health and manage diseases? I'm sure you would want to know how.

To achieve this, you have to eat minimally processed foods. Take in whole foods such as whole grain, vegetables, fruits and nuts and when opting for meat, go for lean meat instead. Drink lots of water, exercise regularly and eat six times a day in the right proportions.

Here are some of the health benefits of eating clean;

1. Makes you feel energetic

A clean diet nourishes your health and gives you the energy required in your everyday activities. Whole foods are rich in nutrients and minerals such as Iron and B-Complex vitamins which enable the access of energy cells.
 By avoiding sugar-filled processed foods and eating unprocessed foods, the body is able to regulate blood sugar levels thereby boosting your health and reducing the risk of heart disease.

2. Reduces the risk of cancer

Most processed foods are sugar filled and contain saturated fats which increase the risk of cancer. Eating a clean diet rich in vegetables and fruits boosts your intake of phytonutrients and antioxidants, which fight cancer growth.
In this case, you can opt for cruciferous veggies - a family that includes broccoli and kale - and tomatoes which are known to be especially beneficial in reducing the risk of cancer.

3. Improves your mental health

A clean diet not only improves your physical well-being but also your mental health which is vitally important for the proper functioning of the body as a whole.

Nutrients from clean eating such as vitamin B-6, help in making of dopamine which is a vital chemical in the brain for increasing feelings and pleasure. Omega-

3 FATTY ACID is also useful in boosting memory and reducing depression and anxiety.

4. Improves cardiovascular health

Cardiovascular diseases are associated with unhealthy eating and refined foods. A clean diet will greatly reduce your risk of getting a cardiovascular disease. For example, fruits and vegetables come packed with vitamin C, a nutrient that helps maintain the strength of your blood vessels.

This also reduces the risk of coronary heart disease and protects you from stroke and high blood pressure. Healthy fats found in fruits such as avocado, certain type of nuts and olive oil, are also vital in combating harmful cholesterol levels. This in turn lowers the risk for cardiovascular diseases.

5. Boosts the health of your skin

A glowing skin which is radiant and healthy can only be achieved by eating the right things. Eating fruits and vegetables regularly has been found to improve the health of your skin and also prevent premature aging signs such as fine lines and wrinkles.

6. Reduces diabetes risk

Diabetes is caused by consuming too much sugar and processed junk food, which increases blood pressure. Making wise food choices to avoid refined foods, is your first step to lowering the risk of diabetes while improving and maintaining your general health. Include regular exercise in your routine and you will completely forget about the risks of diabetes.

7. Makes you sleep better

What we consume has a direct effect to the quality and quantity of sleep that we enjoy at night. Eating too much sugar-filled foods, fatty foods and the likes, will inevitably make you lose sleep.

Sleep is important for your health, and lack of it could prove to be detrimental to many aspects of your life. By eating clean foods, your sleep quality will improve and you can be sure of better health as a result.

8. Leads to effective weight loss

Eating fiber and protein rich foods will play a major role if you want to lose weight. You will control your cravings and reduce the amount of calorie intake which will make you lose fat faster and effectively.

Clean foods also contain necessary anti-oxidants and anti-inflammatory components which are pivotal for successful weight loss. A slimmer body is good for your health in many ways, so you should also put it in perspective by eating clean foods.

With many other health benefits, you can be assured of a long life once you start eating clean and taking part in exercise. You will keep away ailments and boost your general well-being.

Clean Eating 10 Day Challenge – Jump on Board – You Won't Regret It!

A 10 days clean eating challenge is the best place to start on your journey to eating clean. It requires you to follow the aforementioned guidelines on the types of foods to eat. In this case, real food which is not bought, processed or man-made in any way.

Food should be low-carb, gluten-free with a clear emphasis on lean protein, healthy fat and fresh produce. In this challenge, you will prepare the food yourself so it is important to make preparations early by shopping for groceries, and cooking tools.

Follow the meal plans without skipping or jumping to the middle, or omitting one of the menus. As part of the challenge, train yourself to eat after every 3-4 hours, but avoid any kind of food at least two hours before sleep.

DAY 1

This is the first day, so it is important to start the right way in order to set the tone for the next nine days.

For breakfast;

Banana Coconut Green Smoothie

Lunch

Roasted Fennel, Asparagus, and Red Onions with Parmesan and HardBoiled
Eggs

Snack

Broiled Grapefruit with Shredded Coconut

Dinner

- Slow Cooker Salsa Verde Chicken with Cauliflower "Rice" and Green Beans
- Cauliflower rice
- Blanched Green Beans

Night Snack
- 2 squares (1 ounce) dark chocolate

DAY 2

Breakfast
- Chia Pudding with Strawberries, Fig and Almonds

Lunch
- Nicoise Salad

Snack
- 2 medium carrots, peeled and cut in matchsticks, with ¼ cup hummus

Dinner
- Spaghetti Squash with Ground Turkey, Cherry Tomatoes, and Swiss Chard

Night Snack
- 1 Banana, Chocolate, and Coconut Popsicle

DAY 3

Breakfast
- **Broccoli and Scallion Frittata**

Makes 2 servings

Lunch

- **Leftover Roasted Vegetables with Shredded Chicken, Parsley, and Lemon**

Makes 1 serving

Snack

- 1 apple with 10 raw, unsalted almonds *(20 for men)*

Dinner

- **Pan Roasted Salmon with Garlicky Swiss Chard and Cauliflower "Rice"**

Makes 1 serving

Day 3 night snack

Hot Chocolate: In a small saucepan or the microwave, heat 1 cup unsweetened
Almond milk with 1 square (½ ounce) dark chocolate (at least 70% cocoa).

DAY 4

Breakfast

- Chocolate, Banana, and Almond Milk Smoothie
  Makes 1 serving

Lunch

- Broccoli and Scallion Frittata with Grapefruit Wedges

Snack

- **½ English cucumber,** sliced, with **¼ cup hummus**

Dinner

- Leftover Slow Cooker Chicken with Roasted Leeks, Radishes, and Carrots
- Roasted Leeks, Radishes, and Carrots
  Makes 2 servings
- Paprika Roasted Chickpeas
  Makes 2 servings

Night Snack

- Mango Sorbet with Shredded Coconut

Makes 2 servings

DAY 5

Breakfast
- Chia Pudding with Blackberries, Coconut and Pistachios
Makes 1 serving

Lunch
- Roasted Spring Vegetable Salad with Chickpeas
Makes 1 serving

Snack
- 1 pear with 1 tablespoon natural, unsalted almond butter

Dinner
- Spaghetti Squash with Spinach, Parmesan, and a Fried Egg
Makes 1 serving

Night Snack
- 1 Banana, Chocolate, and Coconut Popsicle

DAY 6

Breakfast
- Strawberry Banana Smoothie
Makes 1 serving

Lunch
- Carrot Ribbon Salad with Chickpeas, Figs, and Pistachios in Cider Vinaigrette
Makes 1 serving

Snack
- ½ English cucumber, sliced in matchsticks, with 1 hard-boiled egg *(men, eat 2 eggs)*

Dinner
- Collard Wrapped Turkey Burger
Makes 1 serving

Night Snack
- Coconut and Pistachio Stuffed Dates

DAY 7

Breakfast

- Coconut, Pineapple, and Avocado Smoothie
Makes 1 serving

Lunch
- Eggs and Sweet Potato Soldiers, Roasted Tomatoes, and Kale Salad
Makes 1 serving

Snack
- 1 cup blackberries with 20 raw, unsalted pistachios *(40 for men)*

Dinner
- Shrimp and Snow Pea Stir Fry with Cauliflower "Rice"
- Shrimp and Snow Pea Stir Fry
Makes 1 serving
Night Snack
- 1 apple with 1 tablespoon natural, unsalted almond butter

DAY 8

Breakfast
- Baked Eggs in Garlicky Collard Greens and Sweet Potatoes
Makes 1 serving

Lunch
- White Bean, Cucumber, and Tomato Salad with Herbs and Ginger Lemon
Vinaigrette
Makes 1 serving

Snack
- 1 cup blueberries with 20 raw, unsalted pistachios *(40 for men)*

Dinner
- Roast Pork Loin and Butternut Squash with Grapefruit and Arugula Salad
Makes 3 servings

Night Snack
2 squares (1 ounce) dark chocolate *(at least 70% cocoa)*

DAY 9

Breakfast

  - 2 Roasted Pepper, Cheddar Cheese, and Spinach Egg Muffins (men, 3 egg muffins)

Lunch
  - Kale Salad with Butternut Squash, White Beans, and Cider Vinaigrette
  Makes 1 serving

Snack
  - ½ English cucumber , cut in 1/2 inch slices and drizzled with 12 teaspoons
Ginger lemon juice

Dinner
  - Single Skillet Chicken Thighs with Asparagus and Red Pepper
Makes 1 serving plus

Night Snack
  - Broiled Grapefruit with Shredded Coconut
Makes 1 serving

DAY 10

Breakfast
  - AB&J Smoothie
Makes 1 serving

Lunch
  - Pork Loin, Asparagus and Cauliflower "Rice" Bowl
Makes 1 serving

Snack
  - ½ avocado with a squeeze of lime and a sprinkle of salt

Dinner
  - Baked Eggs In Butternut Squash and Spinach
Makes 1 serving

Night Snack
  - 2 dried Turkish figs with 1 ounce sharp cheddar

Eating clean is very much part of a healthy lifestyle and it plays an important role in the general wellbeing of your body and your mind. For everybody out there who has not yet considered changing their eating habits, it is always the best option to do it early before things turn sour.

The numerous health benefits of eating clean have far reaching effects to other aspects of your life such as weight management and coping with anxiety and depression. So many people suffer from depression and anxiety and little do they know that they can solve this problem starting from their kitchen and being mindful of what they eat.

Eating the right foods has also been found to improve your memory which is also linked with increased creativity and levels of productivity.

This report has shed light on all you need to know about eating clean, why you should avoid processed, sugar filled and junk foods, and how you can revamp your kitchen with natural food options. The recipes herein are easy to make and most of them can be homemade, giving you the easiest route to take.

With many of our health problems stemming from what we eat, it is vitally important that we are mindful of our food choices. This will greatly reduce the health risks associated with cancer, diabetes and heart disease.

Conclusion

By following all that is outlined here, you will enjoy a much healthier lifestyle free from diseases and a longer life. Taking the first step is all that you need and the rest will follow through as you master what to eat.

Take out the pasta, pizza and juices and go for salads, whole grains, fruits, vegetables and nuts.

In a few weeks' time, the magnificent health benefits will be apparent and undeniable. Eating organic is always the better choice. So, enjoy the process and live a more healthy fulfilling life from today.

Good luck!

Vanessa J. Hunt

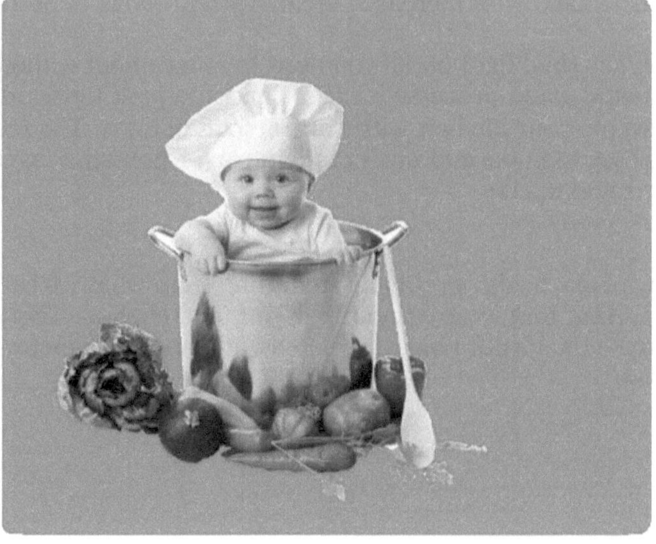

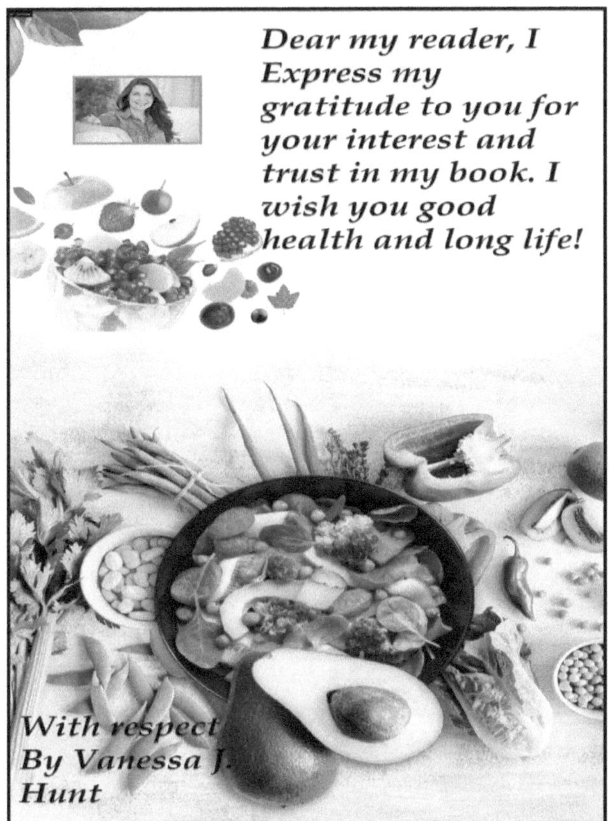
Dear my reader, I
Express my
gratitude to you for
your interest and
trust in my book. I
wish you good
health and long life!

With respect
By Vanessa J.
Hunt